Coping with Cancer

Coping with Cancer

How to Fight Cancer with
Vitamins, Minerals and Diet

by
John L. Sessions, D.O.
and
Morton Walker, D.P.M.

Devin-Adair, Publishers
Greenwich, Connecticut

Copyright © 1985 by John L. Sessions, D.O.,
and Morton Walker, D.P.M.

All rights reserved. No portion of this publication may be reproduced or transmitted in any form or by any means, electronic or mechanical, including photocopy, recording, or any information or retrieval system, without the written permission of Devin-Adair, Publishers, 6 North Water Street, Greenwich, Connecticut 06830

Manufactured in the United States of America.

Library of Congress Cataloging in Publication Data

Sessions, John L.
Coping with cancer.

1. Cancer—Diet therapy. 2. Orthomolecular therapy.
I. Walker, Morton. II. Title. [DNLM: 1. Neoplasms—immunology. 2. Neoplasms—therapy. QZ 266 S493c]
RC271.D52S48   1985   616.99'406   84-9454
ISBN 0-8159-5226-0

Devin-Adair, Publishers, is one of America's leading publishers of quality books on health, nutrition, and the environment. Founded in 1911, the company has been in the forefront of the natural health movement, and publishes the work of such outstanding authors in the field as John Ott and Linda Clark. Devin-Adair operates the Ecological Book Club for nature and health audiences

Publisher: C. de la Belle Issue
Managing Director: Roger H. Lourie
Typesetting: Coghill Book Typesetting
Cover Design: Matt Berger

Devin-Adair, Publishers
6 North Water Street
Greenwich, Connecticut 06830

EXCELLENCE, SINCE 1911

Important Legal Notice

Devin-Adair, Publishers, does not in any way endorse or recommend the data presented in this book. We act as a forum for various viewpoints of different individuals.

We do not necessarily agree or disagree with the material contained herein. This book is published for information and education purposes only. Our books seek only to make people aware of their health needs.

If anyone decides to use any data found in this book, that decision rests completely with that person and his doctor.

Furthermore, any action or decision taken by any reader concerning which therapies to follow or not to follow again rests solely with that reader and his doctor.

This book is not a substitute for personal medical supervision by qualified professional personnel. People with health problems should consult their physicians.

Neither Devin-Adair nor the authors of this book can recommend therapies, drugs or medical courses of action to the reader. We can only alert you to the availability of various treatments and urge that you discuss your case with your physician.

About the Authors

John L. Sessions, D.O., is the founder of the Jasper Medical Center in Kirbyville, Texas, where he has practiced medicine for the last eight years. He has administered chelation therapy for approximately four years, with great success.

Dr. Sessions graduated as a Doctor of Osteopathy from Texas College of Osteopathic Medicine and interned at Dallas Osteopathic Hospital.

He is a member of the American Osteopathic Association, American Academy of Osteopathy, the Metabolic Research Foundation, the International Academy of Preventive Medicine, the American College of General Practitioners, the National Board of Directors of the American Academy of Medical Preventics, the District XII Osteopathic Medical Society, a Diplomat and Member of the National Board of Directors of the American Board of Chelation Therapy, and a Federal Aviation Medical Examiner.

* * *

Morton Walker, D.P.M., is a full time, freelance medical journalist, author of 35 books and numerous medical journal articles. He is the recipient of more than 20 awards, including the Orthomolecular Award, presented in 1981 by the Institute of Preventive Medicine, and the 1979 Humanitarian Award of the American Academy of Medical Preventics for "informing the American public on alternative methods of healing."

Dr. Walker's latest book is *DMSO: The New Healing Power* (Devin-Adair, Publishers, Greenwich, Conn), which incorporates all the known facts surrounding the controversial drug, DMSO.

CONTENTS

1. Coping with Cancer: Prologue — 1
2. What Are Metabolic Cancer Therapies? — 2
3. Causes of Cellular Malignancy — 4
4. The Cancer Establishment Begins to Use Metabolic Therapies — 6
5. Nutritional Therapy for Cancer — 8
6. Protocols of Metabolic Cancer Therapies — 10
7. The Case of Thurman J. Patrick — 12
8. The Manner Metabolic Cancer Program — 17
9. Hematoxylon and DMSO — 20
10. The Case of John E. Rice — 21
11. Building Up the Immune System — 24
12. The Seven-Day Detoxification Program — 28
13. Pretreatment Clinical and Laboratory Testing — 31
14. New Horizons in Cancer Therapy — 33

COPING WITH CANCER

Prologue

When a 1983 survey asked almost 2,000 adult Americans what they fear the most, 65 percent responded, "getting cancer." Robert A. Good, M.D., now chief of Cancer Research, Oklahoma Medical Research Foundation, Oklahoma City, and former Director of the Memorial Sloan-Kettering Cancer Hospital, New York City, points out, "This dread disease is the number two killer in the United States." (Heart disease is number one.)

In 1981, in the U.S., over 420,000 cancer victims died and another 800,000 Americans contracted the disease. In 1982 and 1983 the incidence of cancer in the United States was even higher. Other industrialized Western countries practically duplicate these figures.

The rise in the number of cancer victims is increasing in part because the U.S. population is getting older and malignancies are more frequent in the elderly. The progressive rise in the death rate from cancer, along with a steady decrease in mortality from heart disease, means that by the year 1990 cancer will probably replace heart attack as the leading cause of death in North America.

All of us now face the very real possibility of getting cancer. Today, one in three of us is likely to get cancer and one in five will die from it. And malignancy is the number one cause of death in children.

Is a cancer epidemic unavoidable? Does the nature of the disease make it biologically inevitable? Must cancer inexorably take its toll of the population and become the number one medical problem as other diseases are mitigated by medical progress? Our answer to all of these questions is "No!"

We believe that metabolic therapy utilized both as prevention and as treatment is the solution.

What are Metabolic Cancer Therapies?

Because the standard cancer care has done a relatively poor job of eradicating the disease or of saving patients' lives, a number of theories and alternative therapies have been developed. These nontraditional methods of cancer treatment come under the general term "metabolic therapy." In Europe, metabolic cancer therapies are usually called "biological medicine." In the United States, this kind of treatment program is variously termed "nutritional medicine," "orthomolecular medicine," and "holistic medicine."

The total program of metabolic cancer therapies includes enzyme therapy, pioneered in both Europe and the United States; megavitamin therapy, pioneered in Canada, Europe, and the United States; a wide range of nutritional approaches, including trace-minerals and special diet; and various healing techniques not employed in allopathy. (Allopathy is the orthodox system of medicine, practiced in the United States, in which drugs are used to counteract and alleviate the symptoms of disease.)

Because of ignorance, closed mindedness, maliciousness, or the fear of competition, organized American medicine denigrates health care professionals who utilize alternate forms of healing, which are usually non-allopathic and may include homeopathic, osteopathic, naturopathic, naprapathic, herbal, chiropractic, nutritional, or other methods not employing drugs.

The explosive controversy in the U.S. over amygdalin (Laetrile or nitriloside) has probably been the catalyst for the bitter feelings of establishment medicine toward metabolic cancer care. The use of Laetrile surely is non-traditional. Since some medical practitioners of general metabolic programs also use Laetrile, all the non-traditional metabolic therapies have been lumped together by establishment medicine as "quackery."

Unlike traditional cancer treatments (surgery, radiotherapy, and chemotherapy) none of the metabolic cancer therapies causes new cancers or either short term or long term side effects. These therapies are non-toxic. And where establishment remedies are mostly directed to specific tumor sites, non-traditional procedures attempt to raise the cancer patient's immune system so that the body can fight off the disease on its own.

The essential difference, then, between the two approaches—allopathic, traditional cancer treatment and metabolic, non-traditional cancer treatment—is: traditional treatments are largely immunosuppressive, whereas non-traditional methods build up the immune system. The two types of treatment could not be farther apart.

Not only is the approach to treatment different; proponents of each therapeutic system also disagree on what causes cancer.

Causes of Cellular Malignancy

Cancer begins when a single body cell starts to grow out of control, subdividing endlessly at the expense of its neighbors, until the entire organ or tissue part is overrun with malignant daughter cells, which in turn divide more often than the normal cells from which they are descended. They serve no useful function, live longer than normal cells, have a disordered appearance, and tend to travel from the original (primary) site to other, often distant, parts of the body.

While they are dividing, cancer cells appear to secrete a substance that eventually weakens the effectiveness of the immune system. The substance forms a protective shell, called the "Blocking Factor," which scientists have been unable to identify.

Thus, cancer's blocking factor comes from a breakdown of the immune system and conversely, the immune system cannot effectively attack cancer because of its blocking factor. This blocking factor results from the immune system's failure to cope with the initial phase of tumor formation, caused by cancer-producing agents called "carcinogens."

There are five general types of carcinogens: physical irritation, accumulated radiation, viral infection, hereditary factors, and chemical poisoning, most of which are present in our daily lives.

Physical irritation is frequently caused by repeated injury to some part of the body or by sudden trauma in a region without defenses against the trauma. Physical irritation can be the "straw that breaks the camel's back" after the body's immune system has broken down.

Radiation is a carcinogen. Radiation from sunlight, X-rays, cosmic rays, radioactive substances, and nuclear explosions, in one large dose or in small doses over a period of time, may cause cancer. The invisible beams of high energy in radiation cause genetic changes in cells. However, you can avoid some radiation. Don't sunbathe between 11:00 A.M. and 1:00 P.M. and be sure to use a sunscreen whenever you are going to be in the sun. Insist that your doctor give you good reasons for exposing you to X-rays.

Through research on animals many scientists have come to believe that some viruses cause cancer. Burkitt's lymphoma, a cancer of the lymph tissues, sometimes attacks several people in the same, small, concentrated geographical location, when, according to statistical probability, the disease should occur in only one person in a million. This contradiction in the norm strongly suggests that Burkitt's lymphoma is caused by a virus. Another example is the Epstein-Barr virus, the agent in infectious mononucleosis, which is suspected to be the source of cervical cancer.

A cancer-causing virus unites with the genes in a cell it has invaded and changes the genes' behavior. The likelihood of such a change is probably increased if the human host has been exposed to radiation or environmental chemicals. Infectious viral diseases are contagious, but virally caused cancers are not. An infectious virus invades a cell, reproduces repeatedly, and causes the cell to burst, which spreads the infection. In cancer, the virus unites with the cell's genes and cannot be released from the cell.

A predisposition to cancer is almost certainly partly hereditary. In families with a history of cancer, identical twins frequently develop identical cancers within several years of one another. Some cancers of the eye (retinoblastoma) and thyroid gland (medullary carcinoma), colon polyps (familial polyposis), cancers of the large intestine, the stomach, the lung, the prostate, the breast, the uterine lining (endometrium), and the ovaries recur in the same family. Other families are known in medicine as "cancer families," inasmuch as they suffer a much higher rate of cancer than the general population.

The chemicals used in everyday life cause cancer. Pollution and its associated chemicals stimulate human cellular change, possibly producing a malignancy. Our high-technology society with its many synthetic convenience products tends to stimulate cellular carcinogenicity.

In addition to the more publicized carcinogens are the anesthesia given during surgery, the chemotherapy used to treat cancer, wood dust, cotton and asbestos fibers, plastic food wrap, solder, mothproofers, water softeners, brake linings, beef, varnishes, solvents, pesticides, fats, hormone pills, chlorine in drinking water, fluoride, mushrooms, weed killers, and continual mental stress.

The Cancer Establishment Begins to Use Metabolic Therapies

In 1971, President Nixon declared war on cancer. He stated: "The time has come in America when the same kind of concentrated effort that split the atom and took man to the moon should be turned toward conquering this dread disease." During the next decade the only officially recognized cancer treatments were chemotherapy, radiation, and surgery.

In 1971, 337,000 people died of cancer—one of

every six total deaths. In 1981, 420,000 Americans died of cancer, a 25 percent increase, directly related to the blind-eyed, ineffectual approaches to therapy the cancer establishment has taken.

Establishment medicine treats the tumor instead of helping an individual use his immune system. In fact, immunotherapy for cancer had no place in traditional cancer treatment until about seven years ago when it began to gain respectability in establishment medicine. At the start of the 20th century, doctors hoped that patients could be immunized against getting malignancies, but such thinking fell into disrepute. Cancer immunization has not itself made a comeback, but other aspects of immune system stimulation have.

Lately, there has been increased attention to the problems of immunodiagnosis, immunologic testing for controlling malignancy, and using the immune response for therapeutic benefits. Such revised thinking among medical traditionalists is helping to bring metabolic cancer therapies a little more into the medical mainstream.

Metabolic cancer therapists maintain that cancer is not merely a "tumor disease" but is instead a chronic, systemic cellular dysfunction. Tumors are actually the gross manifestation of dietary deficiencies, organism dependencies, cellular stress, inadequate blood flow, and free-radical pathology. Free radicals are prodigious amounts of superoxides, which, when their mechanisms are detoxified, result in cell breakdowns. The superoxide radical, along with hydrogen peroxide and hydroxyl radicals, are highly reactive elements which affect virtually every cell in the body. People with cancer have few antidote enzymes—the superoxide dismutases, glutathione peroxidases, and catalase. These enzymes, and others, stop free-radical pathology and are utilized as part of metabolic cancer therapy.

Immune system stimulation, immunotherapy, had its roots in France in the 19th century. Yet none of the immune substances developed inside or outside the medical mainstream constitute the "magic bullet" in cancer care. The search for an anti-cancer vaccine continues.

A general rule of oncology (the science of cancer) is that patients with intact immunity have a better chance of surviving cancer than those with impaired immunity. Although the immune system can bounce back, chemotherapy and radiation dangerously weaken it. Nutritional therapy builds up immunity.

Nutritional Therapy for Cancer

Nutritional therapy for the prevention and treatment of cancer has suddenly become legitimate. On June 16, 1982, an expert panel at the National Research Council of the National Academy of Sciences issued a report concluding that there is a strong link between diet and cancer. The report, *Diet, Nutrition, and Cancer,* advises reduced intake of fats and such food as smoked fish and bacon, whose curing agents can become carcinogenic in the digestive tract. The panel advocated daily consumption of food rich in vitamin C, such as citrus fruit, food high in beta-carotene (precursor of vitamin A), including dark green and deep yellow fruit and vegetables, and broccoli, cauliflower and other members of the cabbage family. These foods seem to contain cancer-inhibiting substances.

The National Academy of Sciences guidelines are

based on establishment medicine's most comprehensive review so far of data on the diet-cancer connection. In fact, the Academy's recommendations are "old hat." A number of progressive medical scientists, clinicians who whenever possible use nutritional therapy rather than drug therapy, not only made these recommendations decades ago but have since been doing considerably more advanced work.

Nutrition-oriented physicians are represented by such investigative groups and medical academies as the Linus Pauling Institute, the Metabolic Research Foundation, the American Academy of Medical Preventics, Inc., the International Academy of Preventive Medicine, the American Holistic Medical Association, the International Academy of Metabology, the International College of Applied Nutrition, the Academy of Orthomolecular Psychiatry, the Orthomolecular Medical Society, and others.

Recognition of a possible diet-cancer link by the very prestigious and authoritative National Academy of Sciences makes nutritional therapy viable in cancer treatment. It will also help bring the two antagonistic branches of cancer therapy considerably closer. Traditional medical practitioners may begin to give more respect to metabolic cancer therapists.

Even more significant than the National Academy of Sciences report is the announcement on February 10, 1984, by the American Cancer Society (ACS) (previously resistant to the connection between diet and cancer) that Americans should change their eating habits to reduce the risk of cancer. Pressured by public demand for the truth, the ACS reversed its policy on the subject. Its new guidelines advised people to avoid obesity, eat less fat, drink less alcohol, eat cured and smoked foods only in moderation, and also to eat more fiber and fruit and vegetables rich in certain cancer-preventing elements.

Metabolic therapists have been advancing these recommendations for almost fifty years, but in the past the ACS labeled such advice quackery. One wonders, who are the quacks now?

The American Cancer Society still resists metabolic therapy programs that link particular diet deficiencies (e.g., too little vitamin E and selenium) to malignancy. The ACS still has not taken a stand against such possible carcinogens as food additives, saccharin, coffee, cola drinks, foods made from petroleum, and meats and fish cooked at high temperatures. How many more must die before the Society recognizes these causes of cancer?

Protocols of Metabolic Cancer Therapies

At one time metabolic cancer researchers claimed that a single mode of non-traditional treatment worked best. Each individual therapist maintained that his protocol was the only one to follow, which only served to discredit all of the non-toxic programs for controlling cancer. Fortunately, this situation no longer prevails. Now, combinations of treatments are the rule, with certain exceptions. Some independent scientists, for example, Virginia Livingston-Wheeler, M.D., of San Diego, California, and Lawrence Burton, Ph.D., of Freeport, Grand Bahama, The Bahamas, have developed vaccines and immune system potentiators. Dr. Burton does not prescribe any nutritional menu plan, though Dr. Livingston does.

There are numerous alternative methods of healing cancer. They include Coley toxins, Staphage lysate, hyperthermia, Laetrile, the Simonton mental imagery technique, the Hans Nieper Silbersee Clinic regimen, the Contreras Centro Medico del Mar program, the Hoxsey cancer therapy and clinic, the Gerson therapy, the Manner metabolic cancer program, the American Biologics-Mexico, S.A. Research Hospital and Medical Center procedures, the American International Hospital and Clinic regimen, the Issels Ringberg Clinic program, the Evers Health Center procedures, the Kelley program of metabolic typing and optimal health, the Revici concept and treatment regimen, Ann Wigmore's Hippocrates Health Institute regimen, the glyoxide Koch reagent, the Linus Pauling and Ewan Cameron vitamin C therapy, macrobiotics, Krebiozen, interferon, hydrazine sulfate, live cell therapy, acupuncture, cranial manipulation, rodaquin, Maruyama vaccines, Bonifacio anticancer goat serum, Crofton immunization method, yeast extracts, the Iscador-Lukas Klinik method, the Hoefer-Janker Clinic regimen, proteolytic enzymes, and many more.

None of these alternatives are miracle cures. Indeed, no real cancer cures may exist at all. At best, one can only control a malignancy.

Included here are what experienced metabolic physicians consider the best of the metabolic therapies available. They represent most of the anticancer services used at the Jasper County Medical Center in Kirbyville, Texas. The co-authors and publishers disclaim responsibility for their effects or non-effects.

Some of the protocols for cancer described herein are not found in the United States. As a result, every year close to 100,000 cancer patients seeking alternative, non-traditional treatments travel to Europe, Mexico, the Caribbean or The Bahamas for cancer care. Well-known Americans, such as Betty Ford, Happy Rockefeller, Mrs. Red Buttons, and Fred McMurray, have sought treatment outside the U.S. Why did they find it necessary to leave this most privileged and wealthy of all nations for metabolic therapy?

The Case of Thurman J. Patrick

Neither privileged, wealthy, nor illustrious, Thurman J. Patrick, a 55-year-old Baptist minister from Spurger, Texas, decided to follow the protocols of metabolic cancer therapy.

"I was found to have cancer in May 1982 and entered the state hospital, the University of Texas Medical Branch at Galveston, Texas, to have lymph nodes removed from my left arm," Reverend Patrick said. "The doctors diagnosed my cancer as malignant lymphoma, and they put me on chemotherapy in pill form—called chlorambucil—14 a day for five days, skip three weeks, and go back to the same 14 pills again."

In lymphoma, a malignant tumor of the lymph nodes, longevity prognosis ranges from a few months to many years. The symptoms are multiple enlarged lymph nodes, weight loss, fever, and sweating.

"What caused me to go to the hospital was the discovery of a big, tennis ball-sized lump shaped like an egg across the top of my belly under my left rib. It was my spleen, badly swollen. The lump never hurt me until I started on chemotherapy; I was then in misery. Also, I had swelling in the glands of my legs.

I was so tired every day that I could hardly put one foot ahead of the other while trying to work," the minister said.

Rev. Patrick became an experimental subject.

In fact, most chemotherapy for cancer is an ongoing experiment using unproved drugs. Of the more than 100 forms of malignancy, only 11 of them have thus far responded to chemotherapy. Oncologists use methods of treatment developed in the basic pharmacologic laboratory in clinical trials. Sometimes they work. Usually they don't. Cancer patients are human guinea pigs in most establishment medical institutions.

". . . chemotherapy has not been uniformly successful. . . ," says Philip S. Schein, M.D., Assistant Director of the Vincent T. Lombardi Cancer Research Center and Professor of Medicine and Pharmacology, Georgetown University School of Medicine. In the January 1979 issue of *Resident & Staff Physician* (pp. 21–25), Dr. Schein writes that "many of the important forms of cancer . . . remain resistant to available therapies."

"I didn't benefit from experimental chemotherapy," said Rev. Patrick. "The doctors took bone scans, brain scans, and they drew so much blood that I thought I would be drained dry. They took my blood seven times a day, 30 minutes apart. What was worse, I felt weak all the time; the drug I was taking made my stomach swell up bigger than ever; I had to sit up to sleep. I never could convince the doctor in charge that my stomach was really hurting. He told me the pain was in my mind. Those doctors were just using me to get their training. They don't talk to the patients very much, and hardly ever answer any questions. I felt like one big old guinea pig."

Thurman Patrick stayed on the chemotherapy

program until June 2, 1983, when his discomfort became too intense to continue. When a health food store proprietor in Jasper, Texas, told him that there was a pre-eminent clinical nutritionist, Dr. John Meyer, at the Jasper County Medical Center, Patrick decided to try the natural method.

The clinic gave Rev. Patrick the usual tests for cancer. His blood profile showed that his complete blood count was nearly normal except for a very low lymphocyte count of 6.2 percent (383 absolute count, when the minimum acceptable normal is 1700 lymphocytes). His eosinophil count was high—12.3 percent (up to 2 percent is optimal). Elevated eosinophils often indicate an allergy reaction or environmental/contact type of hypersensitivity, possibly caused by the cancer drug he was taking. The patient's platelet count was a low 140 (optimal minimum is 200).

The patient's thyroid function was variable; T-4 was high at 9.6 (normal is 7.0–8.5), while the T-3 was quite low at 32. This thyroid dysfunction indicated a probable need of copper for the conversion of T-4 to T-3. Such low thyroid functioning would, along with other factors, weaken the patient's ability to overcome cancer or any other debilitating degenerative disease.

A hair analysis taken 11 months before showed that Patrick was deficient in calcium and chromium. He had toxic levels of lead and cadmium. His manganese was extremely high and possibly toxic.

His carcinoembryonic antigen (CEA) test was normal, but the immunostatus differential (ISD) was positive, showing a 3.5 malignancy potential. More significant, the ISD revealed 4 percent bizarre monocytes and 21 percent excrescences. Bizarre monocytes are seen during immune reaction to cancer. Excrescences, the result of weakened cytoplasmic and nuclear membranes, are an indicator of potential malignancy. Blood excrescences decrease during remission and terminal phases of cancer.

From his laboratory test readings, it was apparent that Mr. Patrick would definitely benefit from metabolic therapy.

Unfortunately, chemotherapy interferes with metabolic therapy and reduces its effectiveness. But metabolic therapy administered simultaneously will enhance chemotherapy's results.

Patrick's treatment was begun June 6, 1983, with a complete metabolic program including strong immune support, vitamin A therapy, vitamin C therapy, enzyme therapy, the anticancer diet, and allergy testing, along with the dramatic new treatment for lymphoma, hematoxylon and dimethyl sulfoxide (DMSO) intravenous (IV) therapy, which we will describe later. The patient was given two DMSO-hematoxylon IV infusions, on June 7 and 8.

When Patrick returned to the University of Texas Medical Branch at Galveston two weeks later, his doctors were amazed at his improvement, reflected in laboratory and clinical testings. They told him that if his progress continued, they would gradually reduce the chemotherapy dosage. However, they gave him the usual full amount of chlorambucil, which produced the most violent reaction he had ever had. He vomited over and over. His stomach ached horribly. He lay incapacitated in bed for 10 days. He put the chemotherapy pills away and never took them again.

On July 5, 1983, the patient had another DMSO-hematoxylon IV treatment and also began taking oral hematoxylon-DMSO, two milliliters (ml) per day, morning and evening.

Patrick reported that after enzyme therapy began he felt a "crawling" sensation inside, an itchy feeling, not painful, just a sense that healing was taking place. On August 4 he said that the rectal enzymes he was taking were causing a "deep ache" in his colon area. Meantime, he was given more hematoxylon-DMSO by injection and orally.

On September 2 Patrick again reported that one hour after taking enzymes he had the crawling feeling, plus a burning sensation in the swollen lymph nodes in his stomach. He believed that the enzymes were dissolving the cancer, supported by the fact that three fatty tumors on his back had spontaneously disappeared. He was overjoyed. Also, his stomach stopped hurting.

"Before going to the Jasper County Medical Center my stomach ached so badly I would tremble in the pulpit. Silver dollar-size areas inside my belly felt raw and irritated. There was pressure pain. I could hardly talk because of the pain," said the minister. "A church in the next county scheduled me for a revival meeting, and I accepted, putting my trust in the Lord that I could do it. The Lord led me to Dr. John Sessions and Dr. John Myers, his clinical nutritionist. Instead of one, I ended up preaching three revivals. It was a miracle! I burned an awful lot of energy in those meetings, traveling away from home, meeting new folks every day. But I never felt tired. I divide the credit among the Lord, the enzymes, immune system buildup, the DMSO with hematoxylon, detoxification, nutrients, and my revised diet.

"I still go back to the Galveston hospital, because I'm not ready to reveal to the doctors over there just how and why I have gotten so much better. They may think it's the experimental chemotherapy that's causing my improvement and I'm sorry if I'm leading them astray. I will tell them eventually that I don't use their medicine."

Mr. Patrick is alive and thriving. His blood profile now shows tremendous improvement. Laboratory test readings by the clinic, confirmed by those of the Galveston hospital, are approaching normal. Just two months after metabolic treatment began his lymphocyte count had jumped from 6.2 percent to 16.7 percent (567 absolute count), and no more bizarre monocytes appeared. The ISD was no longer positive for cancer.

On November 22, 1983, the patient reported feeling exceedingly well with lots more energy and a better appetite. He started to replace the weight he had lost because of cancer.

On January 24, 1984, he received his thirteenth infusion of hematoxylon-DMSO and had another hair mineral analysis which showed a dramatic improvement in his tissue mineral content.

At present Reverend Thurman Patrick says he feels "great." He is in high spirits, enthusiastic about the future. Certainly, metabolic therapy has put his cancer in remission. Although the Jasper County Medical Center has not pronounced the patient "cured," he has no symptoms of the disease. He continues to report to the Galveston Medical Center regularly for health checkups, and those doctors can't find anything at all wrong with him. The medical traditionalists are still taking credit for his remission and continue to supply chlorambucil pills, which Patrick just puts away. He assures the metabolic therapists that he has never taken any chemotherapy since the bad reaction he experienced in June 1983.

The Manner Metabolic Cancer Program

The anticancer protocol followed at the Jasper County Medical Center is based on the Manner metabolic program developed and provided by the Metabolic Research Foundation of Glenview, Illinois. Harold Manner, Ph.D., former Professor of Biology at Loyola University, has perfected a protocol for the immunological enhancement of cancer-prone people. This protocol is administered by approximately 200 metabolic physicians located in nearly 75 clinics in the United States.

After he resigned from his university post, Dr. Manner installed his own clinic in an established Tijuana, Mexico, hospital, the Clinica Cydel, for critically ill cancer patients. Meanwhile, the U.S. clinics are effectively treating cancer sufferers on an outpatient basis.

In an interview with Dr. Manner after his presentation at the Cancer Control Society annual meeting on July 4, 1983, he explained his prevention program in full. "We must assist our immune systems by ingesting only those foods that help support the body—eliminating empty foods that are highly processed," Dr. Manner said. "To keep the white blood count at its optimum, you must take 25,000 International Units (IU) of natural vitamin A daily. Emulsified vitamin A is best, a palmitate that has been broken up into fat globules much the way milk is homogenized.

"Then it is necessary to give the patient enzymes (ordinarily circulating in the blood) both orally and by injection, especially if the patient risks getting cancer because there is a family history of it," he said.

"Glandulars are particularly important, as they contain in active form all the gland's vital elements, including hormones. As part of a prevention program, physicians following the protocol of the Metabolic Research Foundation use raw thymus gland, providing its protein component remains intact.

"Metabolic Research Foundation doctors use megadoses of vitamins—especially vitamin C. I think that everyone should take at least four to five grams of vitamin C daily. The B complex vitamins in 150 mg dosages are mandatory, except for folic acid and vitamin B-12 which require microgram dosages," the doctor added. "Don't supplement with vitamin D because you get enough D in regular food. Lecithin and 1200 IU of vitamin E are important; so is a multiple mineral tablet taken every day.

"I advise detoxification with enemas, especially coffee enemas. Clean the bowel for several days until bowel movements occur normally," said Dr. Manner. "I believe every family should have a vegetable juice extractor and drink raw fresh vegetable juice every day, a minimum of two glasses.

"Improve the diet by adding good, natural whole foods and fiber foods," he said. "The anticancer diet is fairly rich in grains containing amygdalin. The diet should include flax, millet, buckwheat, and non-citrus fruits. Eat seeds. Take eight or 10 apricot kernels daily.

"In cancer therapy, during the first 21 days we take away all dairy products, red meat, canned goods, white flour and all white flour products. Refined sugar and all food additives such as preservatives, colorings, flavorings, foaming agents, and other artificial ingredients are taboo," Dr. Manner said. "The typical American diet is a pro-cancer diet. One can eat anything not strictly prohibited and as much as desired on the anticancer diet, but make sure the food is as natural as possible.

"It takes a nutrition-oriented doctor to help cancer patients readjust their lives. But what a difference it makes to them in a relatively short period. In the first week they know that their bodies are getting better."

Hematoxylon and DMSO

A 75-year-old farmer named Marvin Hodge of Vidor, Texas, was examined at the Jasper County Medical Center on October 13, 1983. Mr. Hodge complained of "cancer on my nose," and examination verified that he had a squamous cell carcinoma. Three years previously he had extensive surgical reconstruction of the bridge and lower portion of his nose because of skin cancer. Now, the cancer had spread to the junction where his original skin line met the grafted skin on his nose.

Hodge was given a new remedy—DMSO in combination with hematoxylon—and instructed to apply it daily to the cancerous areas of his nose. Two weeks later, the cancerous areas had turned black. The squamous cell carcinoma slowly began to shrink.

By January 2, 1984, when the patient was reexamined, the cancer was approximately 90 percent gone. The DMSO-hematoxylon solution was doing a magnificent job of healing. The only cancerous areas that remained were tiny spots on the tip of the nose and a small area on the upper right side of the bridge. Therapy was continued until the skin cancer was completely gone. Mr. Hodge did not have to have his nose removed; he was saved by the new remedy.

This experimental anticancer treatment was developed by Eli Jordon Tucker, Jr., M.D. (now deceased) of Houston, Texas. In addition to its effect on squamous cell carcinoma, DMSO-hematoxylon solution is dramatically effective against adenocarcinoma, lymphosarcoma, lymphoma, and such associated malignancies as Hodgkin's disease. Made from a combination of 25 gm of hematoxylon (a biological dye) and 75 cc of DMSO (a chemical solvent), one cc of the non-toxic solution is the ideal dosage for each 75 pounds of body weight. It has almost no side effects and is administered intravenously, orally, intralesionally, intra-arterially, rectally, and topically.

(A complete discussion of DMSO-hematoxylon therapy, including previously recorded laboratory and clinical research results, can be found in *DMSO: The New Healing Power* by Morton Walker, D.P.M., in consultation with William Campbell Douglass, M.D. [Greenwich, Conn.: Devin-Adair, Publishers, 1983].) This procedure is being ignored by the cancer establishment and kept from the public by the U.S. Food and Drug Administration.

The DMSO-hematoxylon solution removes cancer pain and causes none of the upsetting side effects characteristic of chemotherapy. It is an unheralded medical breakthrough which needs recognition so that more cancer victims can be saved.

The Case of John E. Rice

At M.D. Anderson Hospital in Houston, Texas, John E. Rice, age 36, of Beaumont, Texas, was diagnosed as having grade 4 Hodgkin's disease. The cancer extensively involved the man's neck and lower face with large, walnut-sized cancerous nodules. He had extreme swelling of the abdomen and the lower extremities. Moreover, he had congestive heart failure. The hospital authorities told his family that the patient would live only a few days.

Hodgkin's disease is a malignancy of the lymphatic tissues. It is usually characterized by painless enlargement of one or more groups of lymph nodes in the neck, armpits, groin, chest, or abdomen; the spleen, liver, bone marrow, and bones may also be involved. In addition to the enlarged glands, symptoms are weight loss, fever, profuse sweating at night, and itching, all of which affected John Rice.

In April 1983, Mr. Rice entered the metabolic therapy program of the Jasper County Medical Center. He was given intravenous infusions of hematoxylon dissolved in DMSO. He was admitted to Buna Medical Center Hospital April 21, 1983. According to all medical authorities associated with Mr. Rice's case, he was terminal. Yet, after receiving intravenous drips with DMSO-hematoxylon solution and direct application of the solution to the lesions in his lungs, for only four days, he was well enough to return to his family.

Without continued treatment, Rice began to have difficulty breathing and was readmitted to Buna Medical Center on May 1. There he was again given daily administrations of IV DMSO-hematoxylon solution and began to improve. The many cancerous nodules on his neck and face disappeared; the swelling in his right leg and the size of his abdomen markedly diminished. His lungs, which were being destroyed by the malignancy, now started to clear.

With the continued IV DMSO-hematoxylon and intralesional spraying, accompanied by metabolic supportive therapy, Rice once again, on July 2, 1983, was able to leave the hospital unattended. The patient's recovery was so complete that he was able to drive around the State of Texas attending to his business interests and to take his family on an extended vacation.

Radiology Consultants of Beaumont, Texas, issued reports on Rice's improvement. Thomas V. Hinkle, M.D., in his first radiographic evaluation on May 22, 1983, saw that the patient's chest could not be penetrated by X-rays for diagnostic reading because of the almost complete obliteration of lung tissue "of the entire right hemithorax."

More X-ray film readings made by Dr. Hinkle on May 25, 1983, indicated some slight clearing of the cancer in "the lower lobe on the right" lung. But Rice still had "almost a completely drowned lung, probably due to compression of the major bronchi to these lobes, with accumulation of a large amount of secretions."

By July 18, 1983, Rice was on his way to complete recovery. The various metabolic therapies he was receiving on an outpatient basis, especially the IV infusions of DMSO-hematoxylon, were removing the cancer from both lobes of the lungs. Dr. Hinkle reports: ". . . the study shows additional increased aeration of the left lower lobe with the lower lobe now almost completely aerated [holding air]. . . . There has also been further increased aeration in the right lower lobe with only a small nodular area of diminished aeration seen in the costophrenic angle."

Rice did not die from Hodgkin's disease. He lived several months beyond the original prognosis until he succumbed to heart failure. He had felt so well after metabolic cancer therapy that he engaged in too much activity, and finally his weakened heart gave out. Rice died from heart disease but free of cancer.

None of the original cancer nodules could be found anywhere in his body at the time of his death. When John Rice entered the hospital, Dr. Hinkle's X-rays indicated that almost no air was entering the patient's lungs. As he improved, Rice's chest X-rays showed that the fluid and cancerous shadows were totally disappearing.

It is believed that had the man received metabolic cancer therapy before he developed such an acute terminal heart condition, he would have lived many more years free of cancer.

Building Up the Immune System

For a specific disease therapy to be truly effective the entire human organism must be brought into balance. This balance is known as "homeostasis," absolutely vital for the success of cancer treatment. It requires medical attention to the whole person, not just the part of the body where the tumor is located. True healing comes from healthy glands, organs, tissues, body systems, and cells. All parts must work in harmony. To achieve a state of homeostasis, the practitioner of metabolic therapy helps his or her patient in every way possible to achieve immune system buildup.

Located high in the chest at the forward base of the neck, is a pinkish-gray, two-lobed organ called the thymus gland, an essential component of the immune system. The immune system has many elements, one of which generates the antibodies and other protectors that defend against infection.

Another component acts like a cellular sentry, challenging all comers to distinguish friend from foe. In the body's terms, anything the immune system recognizes as "self" is friend. Anything foreign or abnormal, such as a malarial parasite or a cancer cell, is considered as foe. Weakening of the immune system's surveillance against abnormal cells has been blamed for the rise in cancer risk with increasing age.

The thymus processes a broad category of immunologically active white blood cells, called T-cells or T-lymphocytes. The T-cells kill invaders, enhance some immune functions while suppressing others, help antibody-producing cells recognize targets, and manufacture at least four different hormones. A strong thymus gland increases the ability of the immune system to fight off a disease like cancer.

Raw thymus glandular extract and a substance called "Lily Thymus" build up the thymus. Thymus glandular extract is ground-up pieces of animal thymus. Lily Thymus is made from parts of the Easter lily combined with thymus extract. These immunity strengtheners are easy to administer. The glandular extract is chewed and swallowed; 20 drops of Lily Thymus are held under the tongue for one minute, three times daily.

Vitamin C is given in powder form. The maximum dosage for each patient is determined by monitoring the urinary spillover and/or bowel tolerance. An excess of vitamin C causes diarrhea. The pH of a patient's urine dictates whether ascorbic acid or mineral ascorbate is the preferred vitamin C form. Sometimes intravenous vitamin C is given.

Dr. Harold Manner recommends vitamin A in an emulsified solution, which is absorbed more directly into the body without placing an unnecessary load on the liver. The usual beginning dose is 100,000 IU of vitamin A with steady increases according to the patient's tolerance. Both vitamin A and C assist in the buildup of the immune system.

Amygdalin in the form of Laetrile, which the individual patient must get on his own, is administered by the doctor either orally or by IV infusion. Anyone using Laetrile should have cyanide blood levels monitored to assure that safe and effective amounts of blood cyanide are present.

Enzyme therapy is a key part of the anticancer program, as enzymes break down the fibrous coatings and blocking factors that shield malignant cells from a stimulated immune system. They also clean up the body's intercellular debris. The type of enzymes, the intensity of administration, the pathways of application, and other factors play important roles in effective enzyme therapy.

The metabolic therapist uses the highest quality pancreatic enzymes, to be taken by the patient as a regular food supplement with each meal. Pancreatic enzymes aid digestion and assure that the other more specialized enzymes are free to detoxify the body and attack malignant tissues.

Wobe Mugos, developed by the West German firm Mugos Emulsionagessellschaft, mbh, is to be taken every day in enemas. The Mugos enzyme works especially well with vitamin A. Sometimes it is injected intramuscularly for a more general effect, or it may be injected directly into or around the tumor. For physicians interested in adapting enzyme therapy, see *Enzyme Therapy* (New York: Vantage Press, 1972) by Karl Runsberger, M.D., and Max Wolf, M.D., both pioneers in the field.

Also part of the program is the pineapple enzyme, bromelain, taken as tablets between meals.

It should also be mentioned that the use of enzymes for cancer therapy is based on evidence that cancer cells are more susceptible to lysis by enzymes than are normal cells. The rapidity of cancer cell division causes defects in cancer cellular membranes so that proteolytic and lipolytic enzymes have a greater destructive effect on them.

To draw malignant tissue out of the body through the skin, herbal poultices are sometimes applied.

Anticancer vitamin and mineral therapy, in addition to vitamins C and A, includes, but is not limited to, the vitamin B complex, vitamin E, selenium, germanium, zinc, and others.

Free-form, full-spectrum amino acids are added to the diet. Also used is adenosine triphosphate (ATP) for better amino acid utilization and for increasing energy from metabolism.

A drink made from *Barleygreen* powder, derived from the juice of young green barley plants, strengthens the immune system. Loaded with chlorophyll, it contains 30 times as much vitamin B-1 as milk, 3.3 times as much vitamin C and 6.5 times as much carotene (vitamin A) as spinach, 11 times the amount of calcium in cow's milk, nearly five times the iron content of spinach, almost seven times the vitamin C in oranges, four times the vitamin B-1 in whole wheat flour, plus 30 mcg of vitamin B-12 per 100 gm of dried barley plant juice. Superoxide dismutase (SOD), which is in all living cells, is also found in high concentration in this juice from young barley leaves.

Superoxide dismutase, glutathione peroxidase, and catalase should also be taken by a cancer patient to detoxify the cells. They dissipate free radical pathology, an exceedingly important part of the metabolic therapeutic program.

The Seven-Day Detoxification Program

The human body often behaves just like an automobile. When a car's engine is full of sludge and carbon, it reacts poorly when you step on the accelerator. Even though you put in the highest grade gasoline and the best oil nothing much happens when you try to make the car go.

In the same way, the body can't be up to par if its cells are clogged with acid, sugar, mucus, pus, and other impurities. The result is loss of appetite, poor complexion, sleeplessness, dull-looking eyes, aches and pains, nervousness, irritability, apathy, negative outlook on life, depression, and other indications of illness. The logical solution is a "cleanout." A seven-day detoxification program of metabolic therapy similar to the one used at the Jasper County Medical Center gets rid of the accumulated toxic material from most of the internal organs.

For one full week the cancer patient feasts on an abundance of nature's life-sustaining foods, such as fresh juice, fruit, vegetables, and some special super-nutrients. Food such as beef, pork, poultry, dairy products, fish, veal, and other forms of animal protein are eliminated from the diet and substituted with *Barleygreen,* green drinks, garlic, bee propolis, enzyme tablets, "Catalyst Water," and such natural stool bulk producers as bentonite.

When enough of these detoxifying substances reach the cells, there will be an incredible flushing of waste material—toxic stuff that has robbed you of your vitality. It is important, however, to begin this program with clean bowels, which requires colonic irrigation, either with a high colonic hygiene unit or with an "ascorbate flush." Not only do high dosage ascorbates clean the colon, they saturate your entire body with vitamin C to protect against virus, bacterial, and fungal infections. (You may prefer a good bulk-forming laxative.)

For the most effective cleansing, use a high coffee enema every day, even several per day. The high coffee enema stimulates the liver, alkalines the duodenum, and helps eliminate toxic wastes. It dissolves encrusted wastes that have accumulated along the colon walls, and the caffeine content encourages peristaltic muscle contraction to loosen deposits which may show up as "ropes" of mucus. Gradually, as protein metabolism improves, the colon's muscle tone also improves and bowel movements become normal without the aid of an enema. The organ benefiting most from a coffee enema, however, is the liver, as the flushing helps it to perform the body's detoxification process more effectively.

In Catalyst Water (once known as Willard Water), the spatial relationship of its molecules are altered so as to potentiate the life-sustaining properties of water. It has a normalizing effect on body cells, tissues, and organs, and dissolves nutrients, enzymes, hormones and other substances so they may be more effectively carried to cells.

Mucozyme is an herbal preparation of comfrey and pepsin that absorbs the mucus coating along the intestinal tract to better assimilate nutrients.

Benefits may also be derived from deodorized, allicin-modified pure aged garlic extract in liquid, powder, capsule, or tablet form.

Imported from Europe, bee propolis, a natural antiviral, antibacterial, and antifungal agent, strengthens the immune system and works well as a powerful systemic detoxifier.

Heavy metal/excess mineral detox consists of chelating out excess minerals from the body. Intravenous chelation therapy or oral chelation with specific nutritional supplements is utilized for the heavy metal detoxification.

Herbal laxatives are used as needed for cancer patients who do not have the normal 12- to 18-hour bowel transit time.

The detoxification diet is specific for each day of the week. The first day, only fresh fruit and vegetable juices are taken, in large quantities. Use a vegetable juicer.

For the next three days breakfast consists of citrus juice, 5 level tablespoonsful of yogurt, all kinds of whole, fresh fruit (except dates and avocados), decaffeinated or substitute (cereal-type) coffee, and absolutely no sugar of any kind except perhaps tupelo honey. Drink lots of juice before lunch.

Lunch is two cups of vegetable broth, a large raw salad of fresh vegetables, and fresh fruit.

Dinner consists of two cups of vegetable broth, raw salad, steamed vegetables, and a baked apple. Drink all the juice you want.

The menus for the fifth through seventh days are the same, except at dinner you may add a baked potato, one steamed vegetable, and a medium-sized piece of baked or broiled fish.

The Bacillus Calmette Guerin (BCG) injection utilizes a tuberculosis vaccine which elicits a strong response from the immune system so that the patient can fight off the malignant invader. BCG is not used until well after the immune system has been built up to peak performance.

The immuno-augmentative approach to cancer control also includes utilization of the blocking protein, tumor antibody, tumor complement, and de-blocking protein vaccines developed by Lawrence Burton, Ph.D., of Freeport, The Bahamas.

The basic principle governing metabolic treatment is that substances be not only efficacious, but also non-toxic. As in traditional medicine, some of the metabolic therapeutic substances are still considered experimental, but unlike traditional cancer therapies, practically none of them will harm the patient.

The metabolic therapies we have described are not the only ones available, exclusive of other procedures and considered beneficial to the cancer patient. Still, they are those most commonly used for controlling cancer.

The metabolic therapies, tests, substances, techniques and/or other items described in this book should be undertaken only under the strict supervision of a physician. The co-authors and publishers disclaim any responsibility for the effects, good or bad, that result from employing any method, procedure, material, product, or whatever else contained herein. Furthermore, a series of pretreatment diagnostic and allergy tests must be done before any of these therapeutic procedures are followed.

Pretreatment Clinical and Laboratory Testing

Prior to the use of any of the metabolic therapies for cancer control, particular pretreatment tests must be given by the supervising physician to determine the state of the patient's general health, the ability of his or her immune system to fight off the malignancy, and the patient's allergic sensitivity to any of the therapeutic procedures.

The patient's blood profile is determined by a multichannel (SMAC 25) screening that covers all the fundamental blood chemistries, including a thyroid screen, high density lipid assessment, and complete blood count.

A hair analysis is done to determine the actual tissue-levels of essential and toxic minerals.

A telemetry gastric analysis, using the Heidelberg Capsule, in which the patient swallows a miniature radio transmitter, accurately records the pH of the stomach and duodenum. The test determines the patient's ability to adequately produce hydrochloric acid against alkalines.

Other tests are:

Saliva and urine pH readings.

Complete urinalysis.

Food and inhalant allergy tests. The doctor especially looks for masked or hidden allergens.

Six-hour blood glucose tolerance test (GTT) for blood sugar irregularities.

Adrenal efficiency test.

Positive indican test for the presence and extent of chronic bowel toxicity.

Basel temperature test, developed by Broda Barnes, M.D., to assess the functional capacity of the thyroid.

A full scale series of studies to determine the extent of the patient's malignancy. These include the immunostatus differential (ISD), the carcinoembryonic antigen (CEA) test, the human chorionic gonadotrophin (HCG) test, and the Burton immunocompetence tests. Each of these tests works best for assessing different types of cancer. For example, the Burton test is particularly effective for metastatic prostate cancer, melanoma, bladder cancer, and tumors of the head and neck.

Monitoring the vitamin C content of urine. Urine spill of vitamin C shows that the body is getting all of the vitamin it can absorb.

The ER (elimination rate) test to determine the speed of bowel transit time.

It is not necessary to perform all these tests on every patient. As with various treatment modalities, selection of tests is made on an individual basis, depending on the patient's need and clinical indications. Also, these are not the only tests used in metabolic cancer therapies. Others may be added or substituted. The authors and publisher disclaim responsibility for the accuracy or the necessity of any of these diagnostic laboratory and/or clinical tests. They should be performed only under the supervision of a licensed physician.

New Horizons in Cancer Therapy

Earlier, we emphasized that there are many different types of therapy available to the physician who approaches cancer treatment on a natural, non-toxic basis. All of these therapy methods are effective, but often success or failure can hinge upon the particular combination the physician employs, since different treatment forms work better with particular types of cancer.

A striking illustration of this is the case of a young man who came to the Jasper County Medical Center in May 1984 with terminal brain cancer. The established diagnosis was glioblastoma multiform, and several distinguished doctors had all agreed that nothing further could be done. The grim diagnosis gave the young man only weeks to live at best.

Such a prognosis was not surprising. The man had been blind since his last surgery, four months earlier. His head was swollen, especially on the left side where the eye bulged from the abnormal pressure within. In spite of heavy medication, numerous seizures, frequent severe headaches and constant pain were everyday occurrences. His mental capacity had decreased to the level of a young child and he could hardly remember anything for five minutes. When he attempted to speak, it usually came out in a jumble, that is, if he could find the words in the first place. He could still walk and feed himself, but he was extremely unsteady and required constant attention.

The story began in November 1982. While the young man was in the hospital for a routine tonsillectomy, he suddenly had a small seizure, soon followed by several more. The diagnosis was epilepsy, and medication was prescribed. However, in February 1983, exploratory surgery revealed that the cause of the seizures was a malignant brain tumor in the left frontal lobe.

In December of that year he went into a coma and major surgery was performed. The tumor had spread, and now involved both frontal lobes, as well as other parts of the brain. The diagnosis was glioblastoma multiform, and he was given six months to live. When, in early May, his family brought him for a checkup, they received final confirmation of the cancer's triumph over what had so recently been a strong young man in the prime of life. There was nothing anyone could do—and the six months had dwindled down to weeks at best.

Desperate, the family decided to try metabolic therapy and brought the young man to the clinic for treatment. What follows seems almost like a fairy tale. We quote from an open letter sent out in August 1984, by the family and friends of the patient:

"And so began the great adventure into new hope which has not only apparently stopped the progress of Calvin's dread disease, but has restored him to a remarkable level of health, with reasonable assurance of complete recovery. The clinic had warned that the average cancer case took about eight months of intensive therapy before stabilization was achieved. Yet, in just three months the swelling in Calvin's head is gone, the seizures are gone, the constant pain and headaches are gone and even his kidney trouble is gone. He is aware of what is happening around him and can carry on quite a normal conversation. His wife estimates that his mental acuity in general has risen from the level of a three- to five-year-old child to perhaps the level of a ten- to fifteen-year-old. He is still blind, but can [distinguish] light better, especially out of his left eye. Except for the blindness, however, and certain mental limitations, Calvin is almost completely back to normal."

Though this case may *sound* almost like a fairy tale, nothing could be further from the truth; for the results achieved were the consequence of a carefully planned, total program utilizing some of the very latest insight into non-toxic cancer control. In fact, the first phase of the clinic's program to save this man's life failed; it was only after several consultations and a specific change in treatment that the tide was turned.

About four weeks into the program it became apparent to the doctors that the patient was again rapidly deteriorating and that something must be done quickly if he were to be saved. Through consultation with other metabolic doctors, a clinic was found which effectively used intravenous application of DMSO (dimethyl sulfoxide), especially in brain cancer. The DMSO was used partly as a direct anti-cancer agent and partly as a "carrier" to get other therapeutic agents across the blood brain barrier to the cancer site. The patient received an emergency application of this different, specialized approach; and within a week it was obvious that he was stabilizing. This was not all that was done, however; after reading an article by the late Dr. Roger Wyburn-Mason (Cambridge, Yale, etc.) describing the association of certain protozoa with many cancers, especially of this type, the doctors also added an anti-amoebic therapy to the program.

It is certain that had this special approach, especially the DMSO, not been researched, the patient would have died. The effect was truly remarkable, and there is no question that this particular application should be considered routine in brain cancer. However, it does not mean that DMSO would be effective, or as effective, in other tumors located in other parts of the body.

The connection between cancer and protozoa constitutes another horizon in this field. Dr. Wyburn-Mason did extensive study into the incidences and effect of pathogenic free-living amoebae in a variety of diseases. He especially identified the amoebic infestation with autoimmune diseases (arthritis, M.S., etc.), but in his treatise, "The Causation of Rheumatoid Disease and Many Human Cancers," published in early 1983 shortly before his death, he indicated that this phenomenon was also associated with cancer. In the article the doctor cites at least 30 cases where the administration of different anti-amoebic drugs elicited severe Herxheimer reactions, followed by decided improvement or complete stabilization of the patient. The Herxheimer reaction refers to the onset of nausea and/or influenza-like symptoms, increase of pain, etc., brought on by the liberation of irritating and antigenic substances when large numbers of organisms, such as amoebae, are rapidly killed.

In describing these cases, Dr. Wyburn-Mason points out that the successful treatment was especially seen in the gliomas (gliomata), or brain cancer, and bronchial carcinoma. That is what prompted the doctors at the clinic to add anti-amoebic therapy to the treatment of their patient. In his case, a special form of copper was used. Copper is considered the "natural" anti-amoebic agent, since it is normally present in the human body and is vital to many important body functions.

Dr. John Myers, clinical nutritionist, has made an intensive study of the biological effects of copper in the human body, incorporating data from many other investigators besides Dr. Wyburn-Mason, including Dr. John R. Sorenson, of the University of Nebraska; Gus Porsch, M.D., of Birmingham, Alabama; Dr. Carl F. Pfeiffer, of the Brain Bio Institute at Princeton, New Jersey; and the brilliant new work of Dr. Sheldon Nelson at Michigan State University. The results of this study strongly support the theory that adequate systemic levels of copper play a vital role in the body's natural defense against amoebic infestation.

Speaking of new horizons, a recent one in the diagnostic sphere at the Jasper County Medical Center is the Furda Biochemical Biopsy. This test, named after Dr. Alex F. Furda, the scientist who developed it, opens up a whole new world of knowledge into what happens in the human body. From a sample of blood, a series of factors are isolated, including a lipid panel and an endocrine panel; but the heart of the test is an in-depth analysis of blood proteins, plus a separation of the various isoenzymes (fractions) found in the main diagnostic enzymes, such as LDH, alkaline phosphatase, and CPK. The results not only help the doctors know what is happening, but also where it is happening and how advanced it is.

The Furda Biopsy is invaluable in many ways, but perhaps the most significant is its ability to not only detect neoplastic activity at an early stage, but also to locate it and assess its relative level of intensity. The Medical Center has not worked very long with the test, and more experience with it is needed before it's value can be fully assessed, but at present, it is considered to be by far the most sensitive and comprehensive of all available tests for the early detection of cancer.

One final "horizon," is not really new at all, since it is said that it came down to us from the Indians. This is the use of herbal poultices in the treatment of cancer. The special herbal formula, passed down through the generations, is probably the oldest specific cancer treatment in the world.

The dynamic of the therapy lies in the fact that the poultices are able to "draw" malignant tissue out of the body, through the skin. This "pulling" of the tumor tissue can take place as far away as 18 inches, or more, from the site of the poultice. Although a new treatment form at the Medical Center, the doctors there have carefully studied the method and interviewed patients who have been successfully treated.